The Complete Air Fryer Breakfast & Snack Cooking Guide

Easy Air Fryer Breakfast & Snack Recipes For Beginners

Elle Sloan

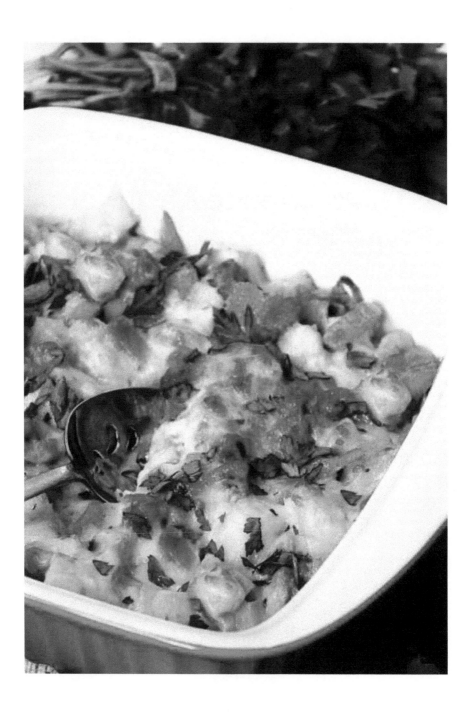

Table of contents

Perfect Vegetable Roast

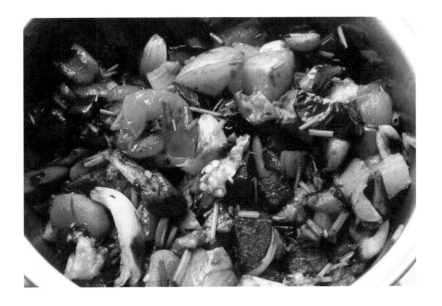

Preparation Time: 10 minutes

Cooking Time: 10 minutes

Serving: 4

Ingredients:

- 2 cups Roma tomatoes
- 1/2 cup mushrooms halved
- 1 red bell pepper, seeded and cut into bite-sized portions
- 1 tbsp. coconut oil

- 1 tbsp. garlic powder
- 1 tsp. salt

Directions:

1. Preheat your Air Fryer 400°F
2. Take a bowl and add mushrooms, Roma tomatoes, bell pepper, oil, salt, garlic powder and mix well
3. Transfer to Air Fryer cooking basket
4. Cook for 12-15 minutes, making sure to shake occasionally
5. Serve and enjoy once crispy!

Nutrition:

Calories 19, Carbs 19g, Fat 16g, Protein 7g

Herb Frittata

Preparation Time: 10 minutes

Cooking Time: 25 minutes

Servings: 4

Ingredients:

- 2 tbsp. chopped green scallions
- 1/2 tsp. ground black pepper
- 2 tbsp. chopped cilantro
- 1/2 tsp. salt
- 2 tbsp. chopped parsley
- 1/2 cup half and half, reduced-fat
- 4 eggs, pastured
- 1/3 cup shredded cheddar cheese, reduced-fat

Directions:

1. Switch on the Air Fryer, insert fryer basket, grease it with olive oil, then shut with its lid, set the fryer at 330°F and preheat for 10 minutes.

2. Meanwhile, take a round heatproof pan that fits into the fryer basket, grease it well with oil and set aside until required.
3. Crack the eggs in a bowl, beat in half-and-half, then add remaining ingredients, beat until well mixed and pour the mixture into prepared pan.
4. Open the fryer, place the pan in it, close with its lid and cook for 15 minutes at the 330°F until its top is nicely golden, frittata has set and inserted toothpick into the frittata slides out clean.
5. When Air Fryer beeps, open its lid, take out the pan, then transfer frittata onto a serving plate, cut it into pieces and serve.

Nutrition:

Calories 141, Fat 10g, Carbs 2g, Protein 8g

Zucchini Bread

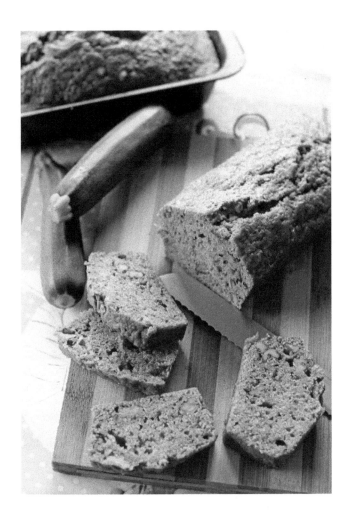

Preparation Time: 25 minutes

Cooking Time: 40 minutes

Servings: 8

Ingredients:

- ¾ cup shredded zucchini
- 1/2 cup almond flour
- 1/4 tsp. salt
- 1/4 cup cocoa powder, unsweetened
- 1/2 cup chocolate chips, unsweetened, divided
- 6 tbsp. erythritol sweetener
- 1/2 tsp. baking soda
- 2 tbsp. olive oil
- 1/2 tsp. vanilla extract, unsweetened
- 2 tbsp. butter, unsalted, melted
- 1 egg, pastured

Directions:

1. Switch on the Air Fryer, insert fryer basket, grease it with olive oil, then shut with its lid, set the fryer at 310°F and preheat for 10 minutes.
2. Meanwhile, place flour in a bowl, add salt, cocoa powder, and baking soda and stir until mixed.
3. Crack the eggs in another bowl, whisk in sweetener, egg, oil, butter, and vanilla until smooth and then slowly whisk in flour mixture until incorporated.
4. Add zucchini along with 1/3 cup chocolate chips and then fold until just mixed.

5. Take a mini loaf pan that fits into the Air Fryer, grease it with olive oil, then pour in the prepared batter and sprinkle remaining chocolate chips on top.
6. Open the fryer, place the loaf pan in it, close with its lid and cook for 30 minutes at the 310°F until inserted toothpick into the bread slides out clean.
7. When Air Fryer beeps, open its lid, remove the loaf pan, then place it on a wire rack and let the bread cool in it for 20 minutes.
8. Take out the bread, let it cool completely, then cut it into slices and serve.

Nutrition:

Calories 356, Fat 17g, Carbs 49g, Protein 5.1g

Blueberry Muffins

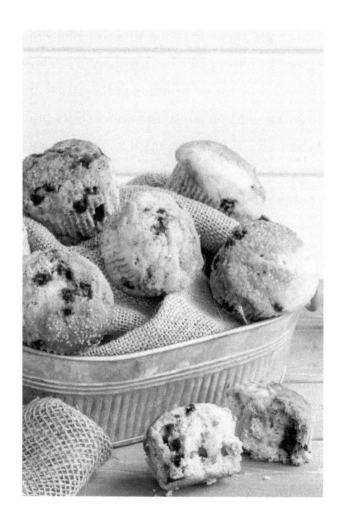

Preparation Time: 10 minutes

Cooking Time: 30 minutes

Servings: 14

Ingredients:

- 1 cup almond flour
- 1 cup frozen blueberries
- 2 tsp.s baking powder
- 1/3 cup erythritol sweetener
- 1 tsp. vanilla extract, unsweetened
- ½ tsp. salt
- ¼ cups melted coconut oil
- 1 egg, pastured
- ¼ cup applesauce, unsweetened
- ¼ cup almond milk, unsweetened

Directions:

1. Switch on the Air Fryer, insert fryer basket, grease it with olive oil, then shut with its lid, set the fryer at 360°F and preheat for 10 minutes.
2. Meanwhile, place flour in a large bowl, add berries, salt, sweetener, and baking powder and stir until well combined.
3. Crack the eggs in another bowl, whisk in vanilla, milk, and applesauce until combined and then slowly whisk in flour mixture until incorporated.

4. Take fourteen silicone muffin cups, grease them with oil, and then evenly fill them with the prepared batter.
5. Open the fryer; stack muffin cups in it, close with its lid and cook for 10 minutes until muffins are nicely golden brown and set.
6. When Air Fryer beeps, open its lid, transfer muffins onto a serving plate and then remaining muffins in the same manner.
7. Serve straight away.

Nutrition:

Calories 201, Fat 8.8g, Carbs 27.3g, Protein 3g

Baked Eggs

Preparation Time: 5 minutes

Cooking Time: 17 minutes

Servings: 2

Ingredients:

- 2 tbsp. frozen spinach, thawed
- ½ tsp. salt
- ¼ tsp. ground black pepper
- 2 eggs, pastured
- 3 tsp.s grated parmesan cheese, reduced-fat
- 2 tbsp. milk, unsweetened, reduced-fat

Directions:

1. Switch on the Air Fryer, insert fryer basket, grease it with olive oil, then shut with its lid, set the fryer at 330°F and preheat for 5 minutes.
2. Meanwhile, take two silicon muffin cups, grease them with oil, then crack an egg into each cup and evenly add cheese, spinach, and milk.

3. Season the egg with salt and black pepper and gently stir the ingredients, without breaking the egg yolk.
4. Open the fryer, add muffin cups in it, close with its lid and cook for 8 to 12 minutes until eggs have cooked to desired doneness.
5. When Air Fryer beeps, take out the muffin cups and serve.

Nutrition:

Calories 161, Fat 11.4g, Carbs 3g, Protein 12.1g

Bagels

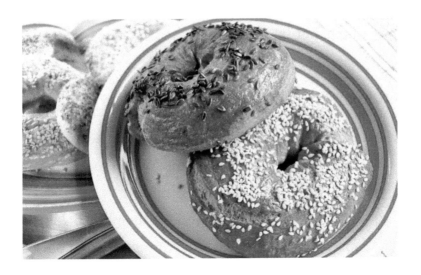

Preparation Time: 10 minutes

Cooking Time: 20 minutes

Servings: 6

Ingredients:

- 2 cups almond flour
- 2 cups shredded mozzarella cheese, low-fat
- 2 tbsp. butter, unsalted
- 1 1/2 tsp. baking powder
- 1 tsp. apple cider vinegar
- 1 egg, pastured

- 1 egg, pastured
- 1 tsp. butter, unsalted, melted

Directions:

1. Place flour in a heatproof bowl, add cheese and butter, then stir well and microwave for 90 seconds until butter and cheese has melted.
2. Then stir the mixture until well combined, let it cool for 5 minutes and whisk in the egg, baking powder, and vinegar until incorporated and dough comes together.
3. Let the dough cool for 10 minutes, then divide the dough into six pieces, shape each piece into a bagel and let the bagels rest for 5 minutes.
4. Prepare the egg wash and for this, place the melted butter in a bowl, whisk in the egg until blended and then brush the mixture generously on top of each bagel.
5. Take a fryer basket, line it with parchment paper and then place prepared bagels in it in a single layer.
6. Switch on the Air Fryer, insert fryer, then shut with its lid, set the fryer at 350°F and cook for 10 minutes at the 350°F until bagels are nicely golden and

thoroughly cooked, turning the bagels halfway through the frying.

7. When Air Fryer beeps, open its lid, transfer bagels to a serving plate and cook the remaining bagels in the same manner.

8. Serve straight away.

Nutrition:

Calories 408, Fat 33.5g, Protein 20.3g, Carbs 8.3g

Cauliflower Hash Browns

Preparation Time: 10 minutes

Cooking Time: 25 minutes

Servings: 6

Ingredients:

- 1/4 cup chickpea flour
- 4 cups cauliflower rice
- 1/2 medium white onion, peeled and chopped
- 1/2 tsp. garlic powder
- 1 tbsp. xanthan gum
- 1/2 tsp. salt
- 1 tbsp. nutritional yeast flakes
- 1 tsp. ground paprika

Directions:

1. Switch on the Air Fryer, insert fryer basket, grease it with olive oil, then shut with its lid, set the fryer at 375°F and preheat for 10 minutes.

2. Meanwhile, place all the ingredients in a bowl, stir until well mixed and then shape the mixture into six rectangular disks, each about ½-inch thick.
3. Open the fryer, add hash browns in it in a single layer, close with its lid and cook for 25 minutes at 375°F until nicely golden and crispy, turning halfway through the frying.
4. When Air Fryer beeps, open its lid, transfer hash browns to a serving plate and serve.

Nutrition:

Calories 115, Carbs 6.2g, Fat 7.3g, Protein 7.4g

Potatoes with Bacon

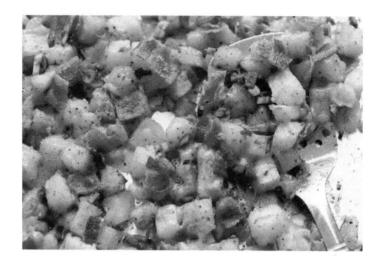

Preparation Time: 10 minutes

Cooking Time: 20 minutes

Servings: 2

Ingredients:

- potatoes, peeled and cut into medium cubes
- garlic cloves, minced
- bacon slices, chopped
- 2 rosemary springs, chopped
- 1 tbsp. olive oil
- Salt and black pepper to the taste

- 2 eggs, whisked

Directions:

1. In your Air Fryer's pan, mix oil with potatoes, garlic, bacon, rosemary, salt, pepper and eggs and whisk.
2. Cook potatoes at 400°F for 20 minutes,
3. Divide everything on plates and serve for breakfast. Enjoy!

Nutrition:

Calories 211, Fat 6g, Carbs 8g, Protein 5g

Zucchini Squash Mix

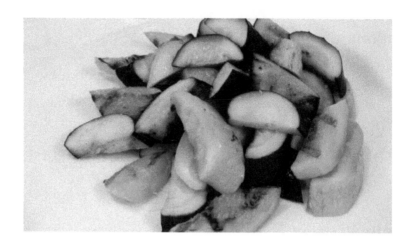

Preparation Time: 10 minutes

Cooking Time: 35 minutes

Servings: 2

Ingredients:

- 1 lb. zucchini, sliced
- 1 tbsp. parsley, chopped
- 1 yellow squash, halved, deseeded, and chopped
- 1 tbsp. olive oil
- Pepper
- Salt

Directions:

1. Place all ingredients into the large bowl and mix well.
2. Transfer bowl mixture into the Air Fryer basket and cook at 400°F for 35 minutes.
3. Serve and enjoy.

Nutrition:

Calories 49, Fat 3g, Carbs: 4g, Protein 1.5g

Special Corn Flakes Casserole

Preparation Time: 10 minutes

Cooking Time: 18 Minutes

Servings: 5

Ingredients:

- 1/3 cup milk
- tbsp. cream cheese; whipped
- 1/4 tsp. nutmeg; ground
- 1/4 cup blueberries
- 1 ½ cups corn flakes; crumbled
- 3 tsp. sugar
- 2 eggs; whisked
- bread slices

Directions:

1. In a bowl, mix eggs with sugar, nutmeg and milk and whisk well.
2. In another bowl, mix cream cheese with blueberries and whisk well.
3. Put corn flakes in a third bowl.

4. Spread blueberry mix on each bread slice; then dip in eggs mix and dredge in corn flakes at the end.
5. Place bread in your Air Fryer's basket; heat up at 400°F and bake for 8 minutes.
6. Divide among plates and serve for breakfast.

Nutrition:

Calories 300, Fat 5g, Carbs 16g, Protein 4g

Protein Rich Egg White Omelet

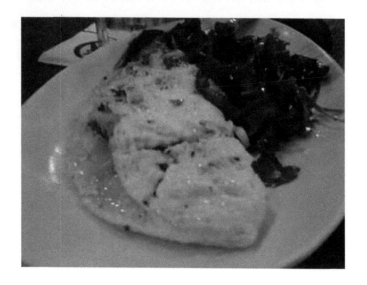

Preparation Time: 10 minutes

Cooking Time: 25 Minutes

Servings: 4

Ingredients:

- 1 cup egg whites
- 1/4 cup mushrooms; chopped
- 2 tbsp. chives; chopped
- 1/4 cup tomato; chopped
- 2 tbsp. skim milk
- Salt and black pepper to the taste

Directions:

1. In a bowl, mix egg whites with tomato, milk, mushrooms, chives, salt and pepper;
2. Whisk well and pour into your Air Fryer's pan. Cook at 320°F, for 15 minutes;
3. Cool omelet down, slice, divide among plates and serve.

Nutrition:

Calories 100, Fat 3g, Carbs 7g, Carbs 4g

Shrimp Sandwiches

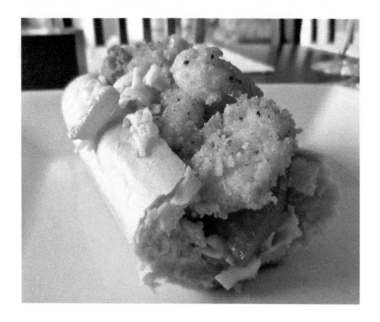

Preparation Time: 10 minutes

Cooking Time: 15 Minutes

Servings: 4

Ingredients:

- 1 ¼ cups cheddar; shredded
- 2 tbsp. green onions; chopped.
- whole wheat bread slices
- oz. canned tiny shrimp; drained
- tbsp. mayonnaise
- 2 tbsp. butter; soft

Directions:

1. In a bowl, mix shrimp with cheese, green onion and mayo and stir well.
2. Spread this on part of the bread slices; top with the other bread slices, cut into halves diagonally and spread butter on top.
3. Place sandwiches in your Air Fryer and cook at 350°F, for 5 minutes. Divide shrimp sandwiches on plates and serve them for breakfast.

Nutrition:

Calories 162, Fat 3g, Carbs 12g, Protein 4g

Breakfast Soufflé

Preparation Time: 10 minutes

Cooking Time: 18 Minutes

Servings: 4

Ingredients:

- eggs; whisked
- tbsp. heavy cream
- 2 tbsp. parsley; chopped.
- 2 tbsp. chives; chopped.
- A pinch of red chili pepper; crushed
- Salt and black pepper to the taste

Directions:

1. Mix the eggs with salt, pepper, heavy cream, red pepper, parsley, and chives. Mix well and divide into 4 soufflé plates.
2. Place the dishes in your deep fryer and cook the soufflé at 350°F for 8 minutes. Serve hot.

Nutrition:

Calories 300, Fat 7g, Carbs 15g,Protein 6g

Fried Tomato Quiche

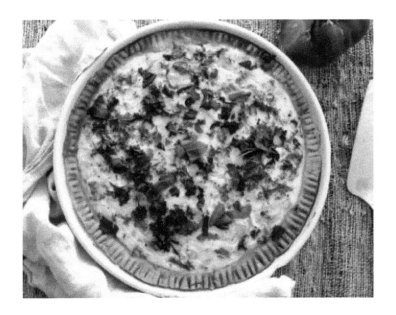

Preparation Time: 10 minutes

Cooking Time: 40 Minutes

Servings: 1

Ingredients:

- 1 tbsp. yellow onion; chopped.

- 1/2 cup gouda cheese; shredded

- 1/4 cup tomatoes; chopped.

- 2 eggs

- 1/4 cup milk

- Salt and black pepper to the taste

- Cooking spray

Directions:

1. Grease a ramekin with cooking spray.
2. Crack eggs, add onion, milk, cheese, tomatoes, salt and pepper and stir. Add this in your Air Fryer's pan and cook at 340°F for 30 minutes.

Nutrition:

Calories 241, Fat 6g, Carbs 14g, Protein 6g

Breakfast Spanish Omelet

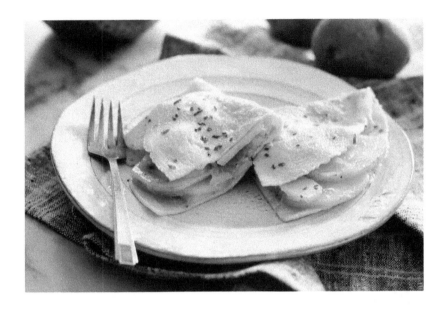

Preparation Time: 10 minutes

Cooking Time: 20 Minutes

Servings: 4

Ingredients:

- Eggs
- 1/2 chorizo; chopped
- 1 tbsp. parsley; chopped.
- 1 tbsp. feta cheese; crumbled
- 1 potato; peeled and cubed
- 1/2 cup corn
- 1 tbsp. olive oil

- Salt and black pepper to the taste

Directions:

1. Heat up your Air Fryer at 350°F and add oil.
2. Add chorizo and potatoes; stir and brown them for a few seconds.
3. In a bowl; mix eggs with corn, parsley, cheese, salt and pepper and whisk.
4. Pour this over chorizo and potatoes; spread and cook for 5 minutes. Divide omelette on plates and serve for breakfast.

Nutrition:

Calories 300, Fat 6g, Carbs 12g, Protein 6g

Scrambled Pancake Hash

Preparation Time: 5 minutes

Cooking Time: 9 minutes

Servings: 7

Ingredients:

- 1 egg
- ¼ cup heavy cream
- tbsp. butter
- 1 cup coconut flour
- 1 tsp. ground ginger
- 1 tsp. salt
- 1 tbsp. apple cider vinegar
- 1 tsp. baking soda

Directions:

1. Combine the salt, baking soda, ground ginger and flour in a mixing bowl. In a separate bowl crack, the egg into it.
2. Add butter and heavy cream.
3. Mix well using a hand mixer. Combine the liquid and dry mixtures and stir until smooth.

4. Preheat your Air Fryer to 400°F. Pour the pancake mixture into the Air Fryer basket tray.
5. Cook the pancake hash for 4 minutes.
6. After this, scramble the pancake hash well and continue to cook for another 5 minutes more.
7. When dish is cooked, transfer it to serving plates, and serve hot!

Nutrition:

Calories 178, Fat 13.3g, Carbs 10.7g, Protein 4.4g

Onion Frittata

Preparation Time: 20 minutes

Cooking Time: 30 Minutes

Servings: 6

Ingredients:

- Eggs; whisked
- 1 tbsp. olive oil
- 1 lb. small potatoes; chopped
- 1 oz. cheddar cheese; grated
- 1/2 cup sour cream
- yellow onions; chopped
- Salt and black pepper to the taste

Directions:

1 In a large bowl; mix eggs with potatoes, onions, salt, pepper, cheese and sour cream and whisk well.

2 Grease your Air Fryer's pan with the oil, add eggs mix; place in Air Fryer and cook for 20 minutes at 320°F. Slice frittata, divide among plates and serve for breakfast.

Nutrition:

Calories 231, Fat 5g, Carbs 8g, Protein 4g

Pea Tortilla

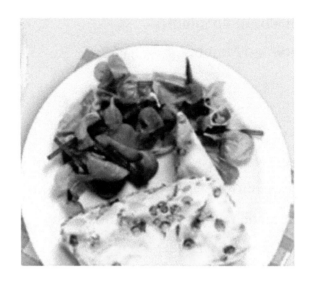

Preparation Time: 10 minutes

Cooking Time: 17 Minutes

Servings: 8

Ingredients:

- 1/2 lb. baby peas
- 1 ½ cup yogurt
- Eggs
- 1/2 cup mint; chopped.
- tbsp. butter
- Salt and black pepper to the taste

Directions:

1   Heat up a pan that fits your Air Fryer with the butter over medium heat, add peas; mix and cook for a couple of minutes.

2   Meanwhile, in a bowl, mix half of the yogurt with salt, pepper, eggs and mint and whisk well.

3   Pour this over the peas, toss, introduce in your Air Fryer and cook at 350°F, for 7 minutes. Spread the rest of the yogurt over your tortilla; slice and serve.

Nutrition:

Calories 192, Fat 5g, Carbs 8g, Protein 7g

Mushroom Quiches

Preparation Time: 10 minutes

Cooking Time: 20 Minutes

Servings: 4

Ingredients:

- Button mushrooms; chopped.
- tbsp. ham; chopped
- Eggs
- 1 tbsp. flour
- 1 tbsp. butter; soft
- 9-inch pie dough
- 1/2 tsp. thyme; dried
- 1/4 cup Swiss cheese; grated
- 1 small yellow onion; chopped.
- 1/3 cup heavy cream
- A pinch of nutmeg; ground
- Salt and black pepper to the taste

Directions:

1. Dust a working surface with the flour and roll the pie dough.
2. Press in on the bottom of the pie pan your Air Fryer has.

3. In a bowl, mix butter with mushrooms, ham, onion, eggs, heavy cream, salt, pepper, thyme and nutmeg and whisk well.
4. Add this over pie crust, spread, sprinkle Swiss cheese all over and place pie pan in your Air Fryer.
5. Cook your quiche at 400°F, for 10 minutes. Slice and serve for breakfast.

Nutrition:
Calories 212, Fat 4g, Carbs 7g, Protein 7g

Walnuts Pear Oatmeal

Preparation Time: 10 minutes
Cooking Time: 17 Minutes
Servings: 4

Ingredients:

- 1 tbsp. butter; soft
- 1/4 cups brown sugar
- 1 cup water
- 1/2 cup raisins
- 1/2 tsp. cinnamon powder
- 1 cup rolled oats
- 1/2 cup walnuts; chopped.
- 2 cups pear; peeled and chopped.

Directions:

1. Mix milk with sugar, butter, oats, cinnamon, raisins, pears and walnuts; stir,
2. Introduce in your fryer and cook at 360°F, for 12 minutes.
3. Divide into bowls and serve.

Nutrition:

Calories 230, Fat 6g, Carbs 20g, Protein 5g

Breakfast Raspberry Rolls

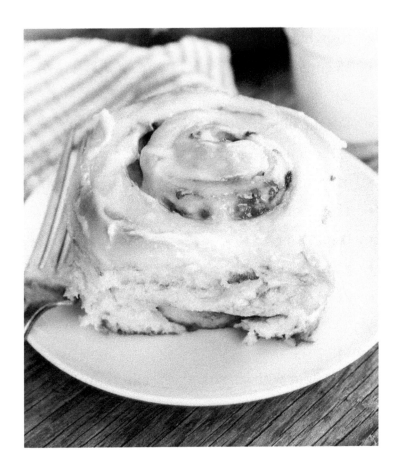

Preparation Time: 10 minutes

Cooking Time: 50 Minutes

Servings: 6

Ingredients:

- 1 cup milk

- 1/4 cup sugar
- 1 egg
- tbsp. butter
- ¼ cups flour
- tsp. yeast
- For the filling:
- oz. cream cheese; soft
- oz. raspberries
- 1 tsp. vanilla extract
- tbsp. sugar
- 1 tbsp. cornstarch
- Zest from 1 lemon; grated

Directions:

1. Mix flour with sugar and yeast and stir.
2. Add milk and egg, stir until you obtain a dough, leave it aside to rise for 30 minutes; transfer dough to a working surface and roll well.
3. Mix cream cheese with sugar, vanilla and lemon zest; stir well and spread over dough.
4. In another bowl, mix raspberries with cornstarch, stir and spread over cream cheese mix.
5. Roll your dough, cut into medium pieces, place them in your Air Fryer; spray them with cooking spray and

cook them at 350°F, for 30 minutes. Serve your rolls for breakfast.

Nutrition:

Calories 261, Fat 5g, Carbs 9g, Protein 6g

Bread Pudding

Preparation Time: 10 minutes
Cooking Time: 32 Minutes
Servings: 4

Ingredients:

- 1/2 lb. white bread; cubed
- 3/4 cup milk
- 3/4 cup water
- tsp. cinnamon powder
- 1 cup flour
- 3/5 cup brown sugar
- tsp. cornstarch
- 1/2 cup apple; peeled; cored and roughly chopped
- 1 tbsp. honey
- 1 tsp. vanilla extract
- oz. soft butter

Directions:

1. In a bowl, mix bread with apple, milk with water, honey, cinnamon, vanilla and cornstarch and whisk well.
2. Mix flour with sugar and butter and stir until you obtain a crumbled mixture.

3. Press half of the crumble mix on the bottom of your Air Fryer; add bread and apple mix, add the rest of the crumble and cook everything at 350°F, for 22 minutes.
4. Divide bread pudding on plates and serve.

Nutrition:
Calories 261, Fat 7g, Carbs 8g, Protein 5g

Cream Cheese Oats

Preparation Time: 10 minutes
Cooking Time: 35 Minutes
Servings: 4

Ingredients:

- 1 cup steel oats
- cups milk
- 1 tbsp. butter
- tbsp. white sugar
- oz. cream cheese; soft
- 3/4 cup raisins
- 1 tsp. cinnamon powder
- 1/4 cup brown sugar

Directions:

1. Heat up a pan that fits your Air Fryer with the butter over medium heat, add oats; stir and toast them for 3 minutes.
2. Add milk and raisins; stir, introduce in your Air Fryer and cook at 350°F, for 20 minutes.
3. Meanwhile; in a bowl, mix cinnamon with brown sugar and stir.

4. In a second bowl, mix white sugar with cream cheese and whisk. Divide oats into bowls and top each with cinnamon and cream cheese.

Nutrition:

Calories 152, Fat 6g, Carbs 25g, Protein 7g

Bread Rolls

Preparation Time: 10 minutes
Cooking Time: 22 Minutes
Servings: 4

Ingredients:

- potatoes; boiled; peeled and mashed
- 1/2 tsp. turmeric powder
- curry leaf springs
- 1/2 tsp. mustard seeds
- bread slices; white parts only
- 1 coriander bunch; chopped.
- green chilies; chopped
- Small yellow onions; chopped.
- 2 tbsp. olive oil
- Salt and black pepper to the taste

Directions:

1. Heat up a pan with 1 tsp. oil; add mustard seeds, onions, curry leaves and turmeric, stir and cook for a few seconds.
2. Add mashed potatoes, salt, pepper, coriander and chilies, stir well; take off heat and cool it down.

3. Divide potatoes mix into 8 parts and shape ovals using your wet hands.
4. Wet bread slices with water; press in order to drain excess water and keep one slice in your palm.
5. Add a potato oval over bread slice and wrap it around it.
6. Do the same with the rest of the potato mix and bread.
7. Heat up your Air Fryer at 400°F; add the rest of the oil, add bread rolls; cook them for 12 minutes. Divide bread rolls on plates and serve for breakfast.

Nutrition:

Calories 261, Fat 6g, Carbs 12g, Protein 7g

Rolled Salmon Sandwich

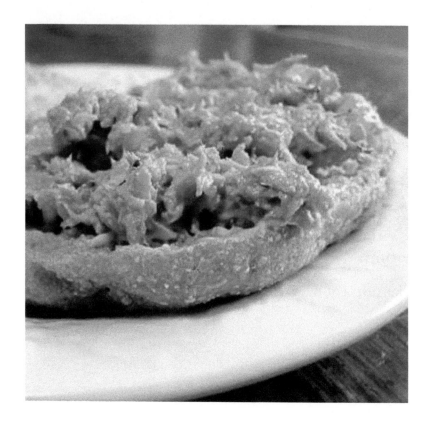

Preparation Time: 5 minutes

Cooking Time: 5 minutes

Servings: 1

Ingredients:

- 1 piece of flatbread

- 1 salmon filet
- Pinch of salt
- 1 tbsp. green onion, chopped
- 1/4 tsp. dried sumac
- 1/2 tsp. thyme
- 1/2 tsp. sesame seeds
- 1/4 English cucumber
- 1 tbsp. yogurt

Directions:

1. Start by peeling and chopping the cucumber. Cut the salmon at a 45-degree angle into 4 slices and lay them flat on the flatbread.
2. Sprinkle salmon with salt to taste. Sprinkle onions, thyme, sumac, and sesame seeds evenly over the salmon.
3. Put the Salmon in the Air Fryer basket and cook at 360°F for at least 3 minutes, but longer if you want a more well-done fish.
4. While you cook your salmon, mix the yogurt and cucumber. Remove your flatbread from the Air Fryer, put it on a plate, and spoon the yogurt mix over the salmon.

5. Fold the flatbread sides in and roll it up for a gourmet lunch that you can take on the go.

Nutrition:

Calories 347, Fat 12.4g, Carbs 20.6g, Protein 38.9g

Balsamic Roasted Chicken

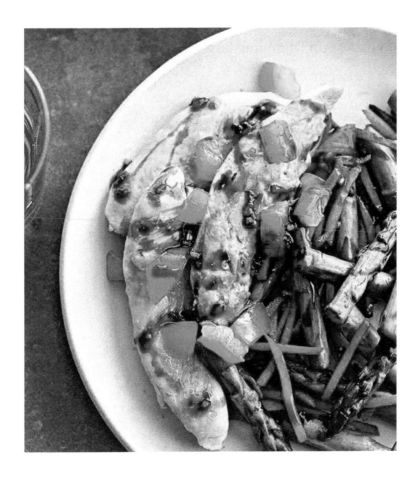

Preparation Time: 10 minutes

Cooking Time: 22 minutes

Servings: 4

Ingredients:

- 1/2 cup balsamic vinegar
- 1/4 cup Dijon mustard
- 1/3 cup olive oil
- Juice and zest from 1 lemon
- minced garlic cloves
- 1 tsp. salt
- 1 tsp. pepper
- bone-in, skin-on chicken thighs
- bone-in, skin-on chicken drumsticks
- 1 tbsp. chopped parsley

Directions:

1. Mix vinegar, lemon juice, mustard, olive oil, garlic, salt, and pepper in a bowl and then pour it into an Air Fryer pan.
2. Roll chicken pieces in the pan, then cover and marinate for at least 2 hours, but up to 24 hours.
3. Preheat the Air Fryer to 360°F and place the chicken on a fresh baking pan, reserving the marinade later.
4. Cook the chicken for 20 minutes.
5. Take the chicken and cover it with foil to keep it warm. Place the marinade in the Air Fryer for about 2 minutes until it simmers down and begins to thicken.

6. Pour marinade over chicken and sprinkle with parsley and lemon zest.

Nutrition:

Calories 1537, Fat 70.5g, Carbs 2.4g, Protein 210.4g

Chicken Capers Sandwich

Preparation Time: 3 minutes

Cooking Time: 3 minutes

Servings: 2

Ingredients:

- Leftover chicken breasts or pre-cooked breaded chicken
- 1 large ripe tomato
- oz.' mozzarella cheese slices
- slices of whole-grain bread
- 1/4 cup olive oil
- 1/3 cup fresh basil leaves
- Salt and pepper to taste

Directions:

1. Start by slicing tomatoes into thin slices.
2. Layer tomatoes, then cheese over two slices of bread and place on a greased pan that fits the Air Fryer.
3. Grill for about 3 minutes at 370°F
4. Heat chicken while the cheese melts.

5. Remove from Air Fryer, sprinkle with basil, and add chicken.
6. Sprinkle with oil and add salt and pepper.
7. Top with other slices of bread and serve.

Nutrition:

Calories 808, Fat 43.6g, Carbs 30.7g, Protein 78.4g

Easy Prosciutto Grilled Cheese

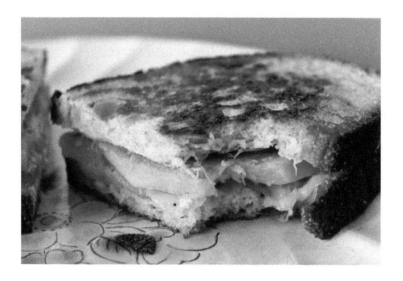

Preparation Time: 5 minutes

Cooking Time: 4 minutes

Servings: 1

Ingredients:

- 4 slices muenster cheese
- 2 slices white bread
- 4 thinly-shaved pieces of prosciutto
- 1 tbsp. sweet and spicy pickles

Directions:

1. Put one slice of cheese on each piece of bread.
2. Put prosciutto on one slice and pickles on the other.
3. Put it in the Air Fryer basket for 4 minutes at 340°F or until the cheese is melted.
4. Combine the sides, cut, and serve.

Nutrition:

Calories 460, Fat 25.2g, Carbs 11.9g, Protein 44.2g

Herb-Roasted Chicken Tenders

Preparation Time: 5 minutes

Cooking Time: 5 minutes

Servings: 2

Ingredients:

- 10 oz. chicken tenders
- 1 tbsp. olive oil
- 1/2 tsp. Herbes de Provence
- tbsp. Dijon mustard
- 1 tbsp. honey
- Salt and pepper

Directions:

1. Start by preheating the Air Fryer to 345°F.
2. Brush the bottom of the Air Fryer pan with 1/2 tbsp. olive oil.
3. Spice the chicken with herbs, salt, and pepper.
4. Place the chicken in a single flat layer in the pan and drizzle the remaining olive oil over it.
5. Air Fry for about 5 minutes

6. While the chicken is cooking, mix the mustard and honey for a tasty condiment.

Nutrition:

Calories 297, Fat 15.5g, Carbs 9.6g, Protein 29.8g

Ground Beef Bowl

Preparation Time: 10 minutes

Cooking Time: 15 minutes

Servings: 4

Ingredients:

- 2 tbsp. chives
- 1 onion, chopped
- 16 oz ground beef
- 1 tsp. olive oil
- 1 tsp. paprika
- 1 tsp. cumin
- ½ tsp. ground black pepper 1-1/2 lb.' boneless pork loin

Directions:

1. Put the ground beef in the Air Fryer basket.
2. Sprinkle the meat with the cumin, paprika, ground black pepper, and olive oil.
3. Stir it and cook for 7 minutes at 380°F. Stir the meat time to time.

4. After this, add chopped onion and chives.
5. Stir the meat mixture and cook it at 380°F for 8 minutes more or until all the ingredients are cooked.
6. Transfer the ground beef to the bowl and serve!

Nutrition:

Calories 236, Fat 8.5g, Carbs 3.3g, Protein 35g

Turmeric Chicken Liver

Preparation Time: 10 minutes

Cooking Time: 7 minutes

Servings: 5

Ingredients:

- 17 oz chicken liver
- 2 tbsp. almond flour
- 1 tbsp. coconut oil
- ½ tsp. salt
- ¼ tsp. minced garlic
- ¾ cup chicken stock

Directions:

1. Place the coconut oil in the Air Fryer basket and preheat it for 20 seconds.
2. Then add chicken liver.
3. Stir it and cook for 2 minutes at 400°F.
4. Then sprinkle the chicken liver with the almond flour, salt, and minced garlic.
5. Add the chicken stock and stir liver and cook it for 5 minutes more or until cooked.

6. Serve the meal immediately!

Nutrition:

Calories 250, Fat 14.7g, Carbs 3.4g, Protein 26.1g

Chicken Burgers

Preparation Time: 15 minutes

Cooking Time: 12 minutes

Servings: 3

Ingredients:

- ¼ cup fresh parsley, chopped
- 1 garlic clove, chopped
- 1 tbsp. olive oil
- 1 egg
- 10 oz ground chicken
- 1 tsp. paprika
- 1 tsp. almond flour

Directions:

1. Place the ground chicken in the mixing bowl.
2. Beat the egg into the mixture and sprinkle it with the paprika, almond flour, chopped garlic clove, and chopped parsley.
3. Stir the meat mixture until homogenous. Then make the medium burgers from the mixture.

4. Spray the Air Fryer basket with the olive oil inside and place the chicken burgers there.
5. Cook the meal for 12 minutes at 390°F. Turn the burgers into another side after 6 minutes of cooking.
6. Chill the cooked burgers little and serve!

Nutrition:

Calories 299, Fat 17.9g, Carbs 3.2g, Protein 31.5g

Zucchini Casserole

Preparation Time: 10 minutes

Cooking Time: 20 minutes

Servings: 5

Ingredients:

- 1 carrot, sliced
- 1 onion, sliced
- 1 zucchini, sliced
- 1 cup chicken stock
- 1 cup kale, chopped
- 1 tsp. paprika
- 1 tsp. salt
- 3 oz bacon, chopped, cooked
- 1 tbsp. olive oil

Directions:

1. Combine together the carrot, onion, zucchini, and chopped kale in the mixing bowl. Stir the mixture well. Then add salt and paprika. Stir it.

2. Pour the olive oil into the Air Fryer basket. Add the vegetable mixture and chopped bacon. Stir it well.
3. Then add the chicken stock and cook the casserole for 20 minutes at 375°F. Stir it gently time to time.
4. When the time is over – check if all the ingredients are cooked.
5. Chill the casserole to the room temperature and serve!

Nutrition:

Calories 146, Fat 10.2g, Carbs 6.6g, Protein 7.7g

Cherry Tuscan Pork Loin

Preparation Time: 15 minutes

Cooking Time: 40 minutes

Servings: 5

Ingredients:

- 1-lb. pork loin
- ½ lemon
- 1 cup cherry tomatoes
- 1 tsp. chili pepper
- 1 tbsp. olive oil
- 1 onion, chopped
- 1 garlic clove, chopped

Directions:

1. Pour the olive oil into the air fryer basket.
2. Sprinkle the pork loin with the chili pepper and garlic clove.
3. Place the pork loin in the air fryer basket and cook it for 20 minutes from one side at 360°F.

4. After this, turn the pork loin into another side and cook it for 10 minutes more.
5. Add the cherry tomatoes.
6. Squeeze the lemon juice over the meat and tomatoes and cook the meal for 10 minutes more at 360°F.
7. When the meat is cooked – let it chill for 5 minutes.
8. Enjoy!

Nutrition:

Calories 262g, Fat 15.6g, Carbs 4.3g, Protein 25.5g

Moroccan Pork Kebabs

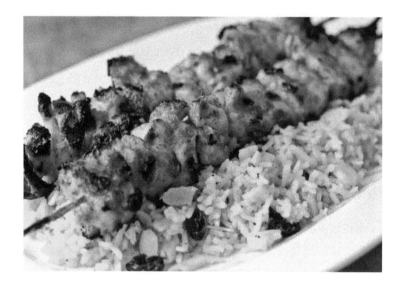

Preparation Time: 40 minutes

Cooking Time: 45 minutes

Servings: 4

Ingredients:

- 1/4 cup orange juice
- 1 tbsp. tomato paste
- 1 clove chopped garlic
- 1 tbsp. ground cumin
- 1/8 tsp. ground cinnamon

- tbsp. olive oil
- 1-1/2 tsp.s salt
- 3/4 tsp. black pepper
- 1-1/2 lb. boneless pork loin
- 1 small eggplant
- 1 small red onion
- Pita bread (optional)
- 1/2 small cucumber
- tbsp. chopped fresh mint
- Wooden skewers

Directions:

1. Begin by placing wooden skewers in water to soak.
2. Cut pork loin and eggplant into 1- to 1-1/2-inch chunks.
3. Preheat toaster oven to 425°F.
4. Cut cucumber and onions into pieces and chop the mint.
5. Combine the orange juice, tomato paste, garlic, cumin, and cinnamon, 2 tbsp. of oil, 1 tsp. of salt, and 1/2 tsp. of pepper.
6. Add the pork to this mixture and refrigerate for at least 30 minutes, but up to 8 hours.
7. Mix vegetables, remaining oil, and salt and pepper.
8. Skewer the vegetables and bake for 20 minutes.

9. Add the pork to the skewers and bake for an additional 25 minutes.
10. Remove ingredients from skewers and sprinkle with mint; serve with flatbread if using.

Nutrition

Calories: 465, Fat: 20.8g, Carbs: 21.9g, Protein: 48.2g

Banana Chips

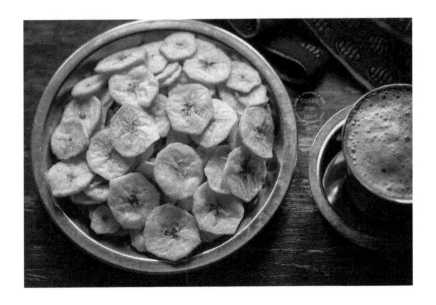

Preparation Time: 5 minutes

Cooking Time: 15 minutes

Servings: 8

Ingredients:

- ¼ cup peanut butter, soft
- 1 banana, peeled and sliced into 16 pieces
- 1 tbsp. vegetable oil

Directions:

1. Put the banana slices in your Air Fryer's basket and drizzle the oil over them.
2. Cook at 360°F for 5 minutes.
3. Transfer to bowls and serve them dipped in peanut butter.

Nutrition:

Calories 100, Fat 4g, Carbs 10g, Protein 4g

Lemony Apple Bites

Preparation Time: 5 minutes

Cooking Time: 5 minutes

Servings: 4

Ingredients:

- Big apples, cored, peeled and cubed
- 2 tsp.s lemon juice
- ½ cup caramel sauce

Directions:

1. In your Air Fryer basket, mix all the ingredients; toss well.
2. Cook at 340°F for 5 minutes.
3. Divide into cups and serve as a snack.

Nutrition:

Calories 180, Fat 4g, Carbs 10g, Protein 3g

Balsamic Zucchini Slices

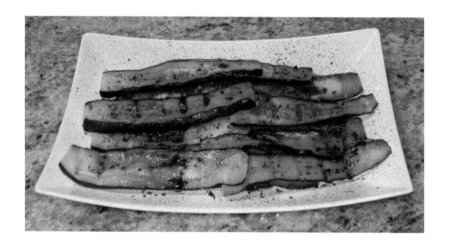

Preparation Time: 5 minutes

Cooking Time: 50 minutes

Servings: 6

Ingredients:

- Zucchinis, thinly sliced
- Salt and black pepper to taste
- Tbsp. avocado oil
- Tbsp. balsamic vinegar

Directions:

1. Put all of the ingredients into a bowl and mix.
2. Put the zucchini mixture in your Air Fryer's basket and cook at 220°F for 50 minutes.
3. Serve as a snack and enjoy!

Nutrition:

Calories 40, Fat 3g, Carbs 3g, Protein 7g

Turmeric Carrot Chips

Preparation Time: 5 minutes

Cooking Time: 25 minutes

Servings: 4

Ingredients:

- Carrots, thinly sliced
- Salt and black pepper to taste
- ½ tsp. turmeric powder
- ½ tsp. chaat masala
- 1 tsp. olive oil

Directions:

1. Put all of the ingredients in a bowl and toss well.
2. Put the mixture in your Air Fryer's basket and cook at 370°F for 25 minutes, shaking the fryer from time to time.
3. Serve as a snack.

Nutrition:

Calories 161, Fat 1g, Carbs 5g, Protein 3g

Chives Radish Snack

Preparation Time: 5 minutes

Cooking Time: 10 minutes

Servings: 4

Ingredients:

- 16 radishes, sliced
- A drizzle of olive oil
- Salt and black pepper to taste
- 1 tbsp. chives, chopped

Directions:

1. In a bowl, mix the radishes, salt, pepper, and oil; toss well.
2. Place the radishes in your Air Fryer's basket and cook at 350°F for 10 minutes.
3. Divide into bowls and serve with chives sprinkled on top.

Nutrition:

Calories 100, Fat 1g, Carbs 4g, Protein 1g

Lentils Snack

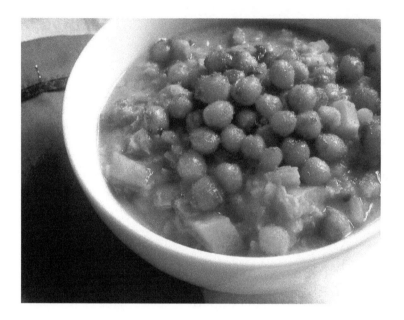

Preparation Time: 5 minutes

Cooking Time: 12 minutes

Servings: 4

Ingredients:

- 15 oz. canned lentils, drained
- ½ tsp. cumin, ground
- 1 tbsp. olive oil
- 1 tsp. sweet paprika

- Salt and black pepper to taste

Directions:

1. Place all ingredients in a bowl and blend it well.
2. Transfer the mixture to your Air Fryer and cook at 400°F for 12 minutes.
3. Divide into bowls and serve as a snack -or a side, or appetizer!

Nutrition:

Calories 151, Fat 1g, Carbs 10g, Protein 6g

Air Fried Corn

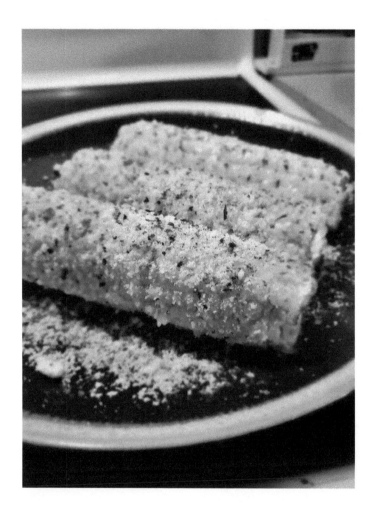

Preparation Time: 5 minutes

Cooking Time: 10 minutes

Servings: 4

Ingredients:

- Tbsp. corn kernels
- 2½ tbsp. butter

Directions:

1. In a saucepan that fits your Air Fryer, mix the corn with the butter.
2. Place the pan inside the Air Fryer and cook at 400°F for 10 minutes.
3. Serve as a snack and enjoy!

Nutrition:

Calories 70, Fat 2g, Carbs 7g, Protein 3g

Breaded Mushrooms

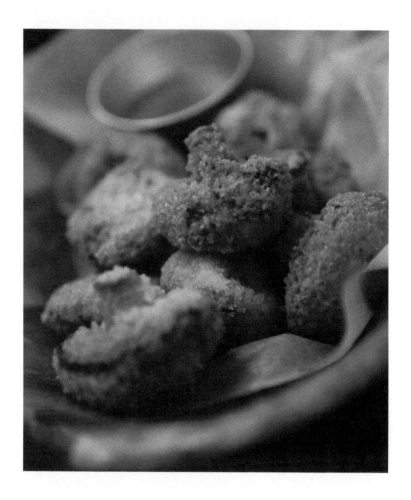

Preparation Time: 10 minutes

Cooking Time: 45 minutes

Servings: 4

Ingredients:

- 1 lb. small Button mushrooms, cleaned
- 2 cups breadcrumbs
- 6 eggs, beaten
- Salt and pepper to taste
- 2 cups Parmigiano Reggiano cheese, grated

Directions:

1   Preheat the Air Fryer to 360°F. Pour the breadcrumbs in a bowl, add salt and pepper and mix well. Pour the cheese in a separate bowl and set aside. Dip each mushroom in the eggs, then in the crumbs, and then in the cheese.

2   Slide out the fryer basket and add 6 to 10 mushrooms. Cook them for 20 minutes, in batches, if needed. Serve with cheese dip.

Nutrition:

Calories 487, Carbs 49g, Fat 22g, Protein 31g

Cheesy Sticks with Sweet Thai Sauce

Preparation Time: 2 hours

Cooking Time: 20 minutes

Servings: 4

Ingredients:

- 12 mozzarella string cheese
- 2 cups breadcrumbs
- 6 eggs
- 1 cup sweet Thai sauce
- tbsp. skimmed milk

Directions:

1   Pour the crumbs in a medium bowl. Break the eggs into a different bowl and beat with the milk. One after the other, dip each cheese sticks in the egg mixture, in the crumbs, then egg mixture again and then in the crumbs again.

2   Place the coated cheese sticks on a cookie sheet and freeze for 1 to 2 hours. Preheat the Air Fryer to 380°F. Arrange the sticks in the fryer without overcrowding.

Cook for 5 minutes, flipping them halfway through cooking to brown evenly. Cook in batches. Serve with a sweet Thai sauce.

Nutrition:

Calories 158, Carbs 14g, Fat 7g, Protein 9g

Bacon Wrapped Avocados

Preparation Time: 10 minutes

Cooking Time: 30 minutes

Servings: 4

Ingredients:

- 12 thick strips bacon
- 2 large avocados, sliced
- ⅓ tsp. salt
- ⅓ tsp. chili powder
- ⅓ tsp. cumin powder

Directions:

1   Stretch the bacon strips to elongate and use a knife to cut in half to make 24 pieces. Wrap each bacon piece around a slice of avocado from one end to the other end. Tuck the end of bacon into the wrap. Arrange on a flat surface and season with salt, chili and cumin on both sides.

2   Arrange 4 to 8 wrapped pieces in the Air Fryer and cook at 350°F for 8 minutes, or until the bacon is browned and crunchy, flipping halfway through to cook evenly.

Remove onto a wire rack and repeat the process for the remaining avocado pieces.

Nutrition:

Calories 193, Carbs 10g, Fat 16g, Protein 4g

Hot Chicken Wingettes

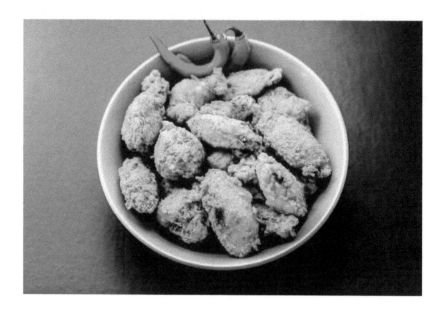

Preparation Time: 10 minutes

Cooking Time: 40 minutes

Servings: 4

Ingredients:

- 15 chicken wingettes
- Salt and pepper to taste
- ⅓ cup hot sauce
- ⅓ cup butter

- ½ tbsp. vinegar

Directions:

1. Preheat the Air Fryer to 360°F. Season the vignettes with pepper and salt. Add them to the Air Fryer and cook for 35 minutes. Toss every 5 minutes. Once ready, remove them into a bowl. Over low heat, melt the butter in a saucepan. Add the vinegar and hot sauce. Stir and cook for a minute.
2. Turn the heat off. Pour the sauce over the chicken. Toss to coat well. Transfer the chicken to a serving platter. Serve with blue cheese dressing.

Nutrition:

Calories 563, Carbs 2g, Fat 28g, Protein 35g

Carrot Crisps

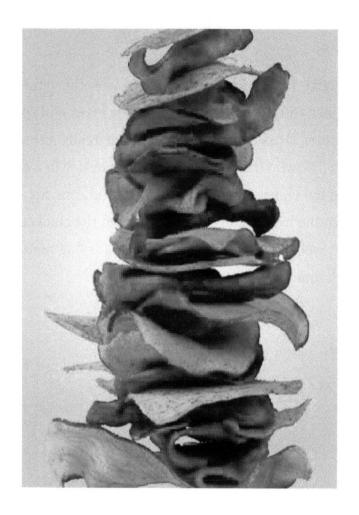

Preparation Time: 10 minutes

Cooking Time: 10 minutes

Servings: 4

Ingredients:

- 6 large carrots, washed and peeled
- Salt to taste
- Cooking spray

Directions:

Using a mandolin slicer, slice the carrots very thinly height-wise. Put the carrot strips in a bowl and season with salt to taste. Grease the fryer basket lightly with cooking spray, and add the carrot strips. Cook at 350°F for 10 minutes, stirring once halfway through.

Nutrition:

Calories 35, Carbs 8g, Fat 3g, Protein 1g

Quick Cheese Sticks

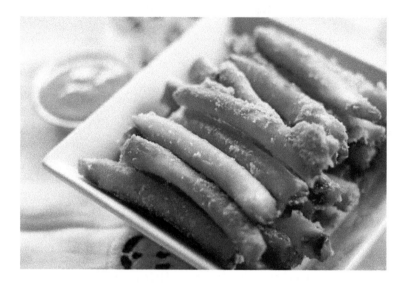

Preparation Time: 5 minutes

Cooking Time: 10 minutes

Servings: 4

Ingredients:

- 6 oz bread cheese
- tbsp. butter
- cups panko crumbs

Directions:

Place the butter in a dish and melt it in the microwave, for 2 minutes; set aside. With a knife, cut the cheese into equal-sized sticks. Brush each stick with butter and dip into panko crumbs. Arrange the cheese sticks in a single layer on the fryer basket. Cook at 390°F for 10 minutes. Flip them halfway through, to brown evenly; serve warm.

Nutrition:

Calories 25, Carbs 8g, Fat 21g, Protein 16g

Radish Chips

Preparation Time: 10 minutes

Cooking Time: 20 minutes

Servings: 4

Ingredients:

- Radishes, leaves removed and cleaned
- Salt to season
- Water
- Cooking spray

Directions:

1. Using a mandolin, slice the radishes thinly. Put them in a pot and pour water on them. Heat the pot on a stovetop, and bring to boil, until the radishes are translucent, for 4 minutes. After 4 minutes, drain the radishes through a sieve; set aside. Grease the fryer basket with cooking spray.
2. Add in the radish slices and cook for 8 minutes, flipping once halfway through. Cook until golden brown, at 400°F. Meanwhile, prepare a paper towel-lined plate. Once the radishes are ready, transfer them to the paper towel-lined

plate. Season with salt, and serve with ketchup or garlic mayo.

Nutrition:

Calories 2, Carbs 0.2g, Fat 2g, Protein 0.1g

Herbed Croutons with Brie Cheese

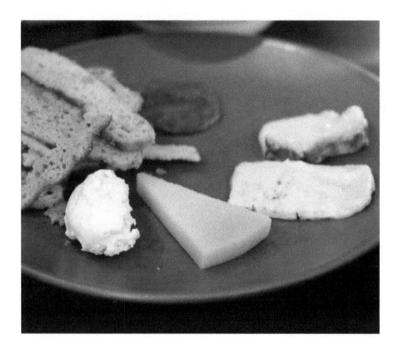

Preparation Time: 10 minutes

Cooking Time: 10 minutes

Servings: 4

Ingredients:

- tbsp. olive oil
- 1 tbsp. french herbs
- oz brie cheese, chopped

- Sliced bread, halved

Directions:

Warm up your Air Fryer to 340° F. Using a bowl, mix oil with herbs. Dip the bread slices in the oil mixture to coat. Place the coated slices on a flat surface. Lay the brie cheese on the slices. Place the slices into your Air Fryer's basket and cook for 7 minutes. Once the bread is ready, cut into cubes.

Nutrition:

Calories 20, Carbs 1.5g, Fat 1.3g, Protein 0.5g

Lightning Source UK Ltd.
Milton Keynes UK
UKHW020629140621
385475UK00001B/40